I0414842

About the author

Alexander Walz had been working for 28 years in the international hospitality industry on three continents before a diagnosis of multiple sclerosis brought his soaring career to an abrupt halt, forcing him to re-evaluate his life.

After leaving the international hospitality industry, he started his own little Café and Bar in downtown Shanghai with his wife and founded a kitchen design company.

Out of his desire to share many extraordinary experiences, he started to write.

Eat right 4 U'r kind

The mother of all diets!

Personal opinions of an only sometimes naked Chef

Copyright 2010 by Alexander Walz.
All rights reserved.

No part of this publication may be reproduced, stored
in a retrieval system or transmitted in any form or by
any means, electronic, mechanical, photocopying,
recording or otherwise, without the written prior
permission of the author.

Printed in the United States of America

ISBN: 1453887598
EAN-13: 9781453887592

For Jenny, Elizabeth, Katharine,Margaretha, Jenny,
Chantelle, Mary, Denise, Cui, Penny, Bessie, Jean,
Bernhard, Adam, Peter, Heinz, Hans, Andreas,
Michael,Gert and humankind in general.

Acknowledgements

This book would not have been possible without all the quirky loops and turns of life. So first of all I have to thank whoever is responsible for this crazy roller coaster ride of my life, whoever it might be!

In addition my greatest thanks and admiration goes to my wife Jenny who puts up with me and my sometimes outrageous ideas for nearly two decades.
For her trust, love and hard work and the beauty she has brought into my life.

I never would have written any book if it wouldn't have been for my good friend Bernhard Brender who convinced me that no matter what life throws at you, there is always light at the end of the tunnel!
Thank you for being there when I needed you most.

May God bless you all!

Content   page

Whenever you see this exclamation mark, I will give a quick outline of what I've learned.
This is how I want to convince you that I'm right!

If you however came to different conclusions through your own life experience, feel free to get yourself a piece of chocolate, a cup of tea, a glass of whiskey, a skinny latte or a raw carrot stick and celebrate the freedom of individuality!
Now go, make yourself comfortable, start to read and enjoy the ride...

Preface

Why did I write this book?

Let's get first one thing out of the way, right at the beginning:

I'm not after a Nobel Prize!

If you really push me hard, I might submit and accept it – maybe for financial reasons – but it's not really me writing this.
Of course I'm the one who is writing it but it comes from out there and is property of humankind in general.

I'm a big believer in spirituality, wonders, unexplainable coincidences and quirky stuff in general.
It all adds spice to our physical being.

For example:
Did you ever wonder how acupuncture came about?
Did somebody sit x-thousand years ago with a really sharp splinter in his hand think:
"Wow, I have this really sharp splinter sticking in my hand and my headache just disappeared!

Let's stick it in my knee and see if my back pain also goes away!"
If you ask me, there is no chance in the world that it happened that way.

So how do those things get discovered?
I forgot his name but one scientist – contrary to me a best-selling author of several books – studies how Eureka-moments come about.
He discovered that they don't!
When great things are discovered, they are usually discovered over lengthy periods of time, sometimes years.
What does happen is that somebody collects an immense volume of knowledge through corporation or observation and eventually all this knowledge is arranged in a completely new way inside of the brain, in a way as it never happened before.
This is apparently how new discoveries come about.

After I read about this, it all made sense.
I am a chef by profession and about 15 years ago I did my master-chefs diploma. I am a very picky eater and had digestive issues all my life.
Six years ago I got diagnosed with an autoimmune disease (Multiple sclerosis) and through observation over the next six years I became convinced that diet is the most influential component of my condition.
I've been through months of elimination diets and reintroduction of food components, observed and

recorded resulting physical reactions and suddenly, one day, everything just fell into place.

I never had a problem with being overweight. On the contrary, all of my life I struggled to gain more weight. I could eat what I wanted and didn't gain an ounce.
All my life, at 1 m 76, I hovered around the 60 kg mark.
Not very good for a successful executive chef!

Now it all makes sense. Now I understand what my problem is. Now I possibly know what your problem is!
Overweight, underweight, tired, nervous, hyperactive, lethargic, disease ridden or just not well in general. Chances are, I have the answer!

I think at this point I have to throw in a disclaimer that I am not a doctor, that I don't want you to give up any of your medications prescribed by your doctor, that I am not a wonder – healer, that I take no responsibility for any of the stupid things you might do based on my suggestions and that everything what I try to convey to greater humankind is my honest and own opinion evolved from opinions of hundreds, if not thousands of others and will stand the test of time!

I hope you enjoy reading what I have to say, make up your own mind and then do what is right for you.
All the best for the rest of your life!

The mother of all diets!

First things first.
You have to agree with me on this one. If you
don't, you might as well decide that you wasted
your money and put the book away (unless of
course you think that it is still highly entertaining
to read).((Or you're a little bit nosy and want to see
where all this leads...))

You are an animal!!!

Sorry, please don't misunderstand, I'm not talking
about your intellect or your psychological
preferences but about your physical composition
(your body).

Your trains of thought is what makes you human
(the software) but your hardware (cells, atoms, fat,
muscles, blood, glands, cartilage, minerals,
vitamins, trace elements, metals and all the other
stuff) is nature pure.

Now that we have this fact established and agree, we can start looking at the bigger picture.

If you do some research on the Internet about the human race, you will find that the human race originated about 200,000 years ago in Africa and we are considered modern human beings since about 50,000 years.

Of course, if you consider yourself a creationist this book might also not be the right one for you...?

I for myself believe in evolution and that we came from those humble origins.

Today our notion of a perfect, healthy diet is the balanced diet. I am absolutely sure that you have seen before the famous food pyramid, which is supposed to give us a visual impression of how we should eat, to lead a long and healthy life.

Even with the abstract thinking our ancestors, 50,000 years ago are credited with, I questioned the fact if they would agree with us. As we started as hunter-gatherers and didn't live in an agrarian environment, our diet would have been very different from today's diet.

Now don't involve me in your usual heated discussions about vegetarianism, non-cab, raw or other fancy diet but I'm pretty convinced that our ancestors wouldn't have even thought about this kind of possibilities. They probably would have

The mother of all diets!

been happy enough to have something to eat at all.

So what is the right diet for us kind of animal?

I am convinced that we need proteins, carbohydrates, fat and also all the other stuff mentioned earlier on.
So what is this guy talking about?
What is the silver bullet for all our modern disease?
What is this mother of all diets?

It is **not**

What we eat

It is

How we eat!

Vegetarianism or carnivore?
Raw or cooked?
Blunt or seasoned?
Omega-3, Omega-6 or no fat at all?
Regular for organic?
Refined or unrefined?
Any or only gluten-free starch?
Hot or cold?

This list could go on and on!

And yes, I know and agree that some of us have terrible food allergies or sensitivities but this has nothing to do with the mother of all diets!

The mother of all diets means that you have to decide what you eat right now at any given meal.

Yes, have the best and healthiest foods available on the market.
Eat them raw or cooked.
Consider your allergies or food sensitivities.
Prepare them in a way you like them best.

But don't eat everything at the same time!

Nobody will be able to prove it but I make a bet with you that when our early ancestors caught a rabbit, they wouldn't start to unpack the nuts they collected yesterday, the roots they found in the morning or the seeds from last week to accompany the rabbit meat.

Our digestive system is an incredible, flexible and versatile part of our organism.
We are able to digest nearly everything this world has to offer. In times of famine human beings even survive on grass and tree barks (think North Korea a couple of years ago).
We can digest carbohydrates, proteins, fats but we cannot digest everything at the same time!

Our digestive system adapts to the task at hand.

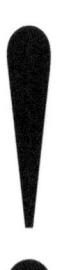 **Don't have a balanced meal, but a balanced food supply!**

The discovery

How did I come to this conclusion?

As I told you earlier on in the Pre-face, six years ago I got diagnosed with multiple sclerosis, an usually non-fatal autoimmune disease which interferes with the transmission of nerve signals.
The loss of the ability to walk is for me the biggest drawback.

How did I contracted this disease?

This is the million-dollar question which nowadays millions of autoimmune disease sufferers ask themselves.

Genetic predisposition?
Possible, but why so late in our evolution?
Why not 20 –, 50 – or 100,000 years ago?
Why is this disease called a modern disease?
What did change in the last 200+ years?

Let me exhibit my train of thought:

Ear right 4 U'r kind

To appreciate the whole reasoning, I will first elaborate a little bit on my condition:

So how does it feel to have multiple sclerosis? Expressed in one word: Lousy!

What are the cons?

The uncertainty what's happening because nobody really knows what multiple sclerosis is.

The myriad of different effects it can have: Numbness in all different kinds of limbs, focus problems in the eyes, bladder control problems, digestive problems, fatigue, temperature sensitivity – especially to heat, pain, balance problems, brain fog, walking problems and possibly a variety of others.
Luckily I don't have most of those, I'm especially grateful that I have no pain.

The worst for me is that I don't have the ability to walk freely any more. Fatigue was a problem at one time but now it's not a big deal any more – I'm not really tired, I just have no energy.

Meaning: I'm not tired in the sense that I want to go to sleep but if I command my legs to move they just don't. No energy!

The discovery

So, no more running with the kids.
No more going quick to the corner store.
No more going to the bar.
No more having a stroll in the park.
No more skiing.
No more visit to the museum.
No more spontaneous visits to friends.
No more work – Huray!
No more feeling of physical accomplishment.
Etc., etc., etc.
I guess you get my drift...

But now the interesting part, what are the pros?

You're forced to redefine your purpose.
You learn not to take simple things for granted.
You learn who your real friends are.
You learn the importance of friends.
You learn the meaning of the words: "...in good times and in bad times, until death does part you."
You have a great tool to educate your children:
"You better eat your vegetables / fruits, or do you want to end up like daddy?"
You can teach your kids the art of persistence – If something you do doesn't work, try it in another way – You never give up!
You become a creative problem solver.
You change to a healthy diet – as a fact, my doctor looks at my blood test results and says: "Looking at your results, you are the most healthy person in this world!"
You have time to contemplate things.
You realize the power of words!

Ear right 4 U'r kind

Let me ask you:

Do you believe in a sickness that can't be cured?
From the beginning, when I heard for the very first time the diagnosis of multiple sclerosis, I did not believe that this is a sickness that can't be cured!

There is no sickness or disease in this world that can't be cured!
We just haven't found the right answer yet!

Even individuals who are diagnosed with the worst terminal illness, predicted to live only another couple of days, are documented to recover completely!
It's called spontaneous recovery and nobody knows how this is possible.

As I mentioned earlier, the Internet is an amazing tool to do research.
There are millions of well-meaning individuals and also a lot of quacks trying to teach or sell you all kind of measures to reverse the progression of multiple sclerosis - to force the disease into permanent remission and turn you into a healthier individual than you ever have been before.

All of that has to be taken with a grain of salt and with a healthy portion of scepticism.

Everybody who does have multiple sclerosis or is dealing with an affected person, agrees that the diet has a big impact.

The discovery

The most famous research ever done in this respect was done by Dr. Roy Swank.
In the 1950s he prescribed dietary guidelines to over 140 individuals and monitored their progression over the next 35 years.

Compared to others, their progression was halted and overall they fared much better. They didn't get cured but they lived a more normal life.

Over the past six years I tried many different kinds of diets:
- I stopped to drink coffee,
- I stopped to drink beer,
- drank no alcoholic beverage,
- eat only vegetables or only meat and vegetables,
- tried a purely vegetarian diet,
- eat completely gluten-free,
- completely eliminated all artificial flavors or colorings from my diet,
- eat only chicken or seafood with my carbohydrates,
- eat no other protein than pork meat,
- eat nothing but pumpkins,
- had 2 to 3 apples every day,
- had everyday broccoli followed by a banana for dessert,
- drank every day 200ml of Gin,
- had every day one glass of water in the morning and one in the evening before going to sleep with 1 tablespoon of baking

soda dissolved into it,
- drank every day 2 litters of ginger tea,
- drank every day 2 litters of Coca-Cola,
- had no other liquid than green tea,
- eat nothing but white cabbage in all different kinds of preparation,
- eat everyday 3 teaspoons of my own medical concoction containing cinnamon, garlic, turmeric, Indian curry powder, cardamom, walnuts and extra virgin olive oil.

Of course you understand that each one of those dietary changes didn't happen all at the same time.

I actually tried one for several weeks and if I didn't had any positive or if it caused an immediate negative effect, I changed and moved on to the next possibility.

Over the years certain principles materialized very clearly:

Firstly, one of the doctors was right when he told me that night-shadow plants are not good for me. Every time I had a potato, tomato, red pepper or eggplant I would feel absolutely lousy for the next couple of days.
Secondly certain foods made me feel much better, one of them being salmon sushi with wasabi, another one is honey.

The discovery

When I re-introduced coffee again, my fingers finally became more warm again (The end of the "fingers of death").
After a glass of red wine I felt great, after a sip of white wine I felt absolutely stuffed!

On the one hand I must say that I started to enjoy and appreciate having an immediate effect on consumption of certain foods. It is like a built-in warning / alarm system. It very clearly showed me that the body reacts. That sometimes a food tastes absolutely great but is having a devastating effect on your overall well-being.
That your needs and your desires sometimes don't correspond.

I eventually came to my own conclusion what causes multiple sclerosis:

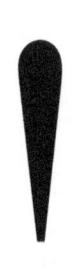 **All the problems and symptoms are caused by our digestive system and it's not really what you eat but how you eat it!**

3

Let me explain this in some more detail:

Let's look at the evolution of man in more detail. I guess, if you're still reading, we mostly agree that we have been around for quite some time. Over the centuries our eating habits have changed quite dramatically. The reason being mainly the increase in the worlds population, advancing technology, food transportation/storage developments and our overall heightened living standards and expectations.

I guess we also agree in general that over the centuries a balanced diet was the exception and not the rule! Individuals had limited access to the whole range of different food components.
I was not there and I believe it's very hard to find out exactly what happened at the dawn of history but I'm pretty sure that our main food source came through hunting.

Now look at other fellow mammals:
Herbivore animals such as sheep and cows consume a purely vegetarian diet and have a specialized alkaline digestion. Compared to humans they eat a much larger quantity of food proportional to their body weight.

They first chew their food extensively to enrich it with their saliva and therefore alkalise it and then re-chew it once again to initiate the digestive process through enzymes which work best in an non-acidic environment.

Where we as humans, have our appendix which in comparison is very tiny, they all have a large sack to aid digestion.

Carnivorous animals on the other hand, such as lions, have a specialized acidic digestion. They don't chew their food but gulp it down in big chunks.

It seems that because of our small appendix we are not able to extract enough proteins out of vegetable plants alone, however we developed into a direction where our digestive system became good at what you could call "multitasking".

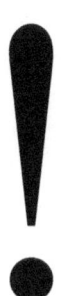 **The human digestive
system is able to apply
an acidic process or an
alkaline process,
depending on the
input!**

In both cases it works perfectly fine - unfortunately
not simultaneously at the same time!
I am a chef by profession, eat food since 44 years,
am inquisitive, rate myself as one of the medium-
intelligent people in this world and love to read.
However in all the years preceding my diagnosis I
never have heard anything about this fact.

Since over six years I'm seeing doctors with my condition and not once has anyone suggested that the way I combined my food might be wrong!

Sure, some of them told me that I can't eat any red meat, others that I can't eat any food from the sea, only river fish, The next one said definitely no chicken – only pork.
I sometimes joke that if I would have listened to all of them I couldn't eat anything any more!

So, let's get back to proper digestion:

If food enters your mouth, your body will know which process to initiate.

- If carbohydrates are detected the saliva will automatically start to excrete amylase, an enzyme which begins to break down complex carbohydrates.

The functionality of amylase is inhibited in an acidic environment.

- If meat is detected, the body automatically initiates an acidic digestion.

Therefore it's of utmost importance that proteins and carbohydrates are consumed separately!

The detailed explanation

If you're very healthy and have a very strong digestive system, it still might work but you put your body under an immense unnecessary strain.

Digestion of proteins takes normally 3 to 4 hours. The digestion of carbohydrates takes equally 3 to 4 hours. However, if both are consumed at the same time, the duration might extend to 10 to 12 hours!

The big problem here is the incomplete breakdown - in most cases - of the components and even worse is the possibility of putrefying the whole intestinal environment.

Fermentation can occur and a large amount of toxins can reach the bloodstream, eventually leading to the breakdown of the immune system!

To prevent all this from happening, it is of utmost importance, as mentioned before to consume proteins and carbohydrates at different times!

Our forefathers knew about this long before I ever heard anything about it.

Even in the Bible is written that God said: "In the evening I give you flesh and in the morning you can feed yourself with bread."

You will find rules for eating in the Jewish Torah, in the Arabic Koran, The ancient medical teachings of India "Aryuveda" with very specific dietary rules, etc.,etc.

Eat right 4 U'r kind

Buddhists eat strictly vegetarian and I'm sure the list goes on and on...

I think it's rather intriguing that the first case of multiple sclerosis is recorded in the late 18th century. Around the time of the Industrial Revolution when technologies made great leaps to propel us into the modern world.

It's also very interesting to note that in the last couple of decades there was an exponential increase in not only multiple sclerosis but also Alzheimer's disease, Parkinson's disease, the explosive multiplication of cancers, attention deficit syndrome, all the other autoimmune disease, the increase in diabetes and any of the other modern-day disease you can think of...

Is it because now it's the norm to eat carbohydrates and proteins at the same meal, every meal?

Bacon and eggs with bread for breakfast.
Lunch or dinner some combination of proteins and carbohydrates. Let me give you some examples: Hamburger, spaghetti with meatballs, steak with potato chips, Meat lovers pizza, turkey sandwich, and the list could go on and on...

Even for me, being a traditionally Western-style trained chef, it is nearly unimaginable to eat in a different way.

The detailed explanation

In the past I learned that every meal should have carbohydrates, proteins and vegetables!

Remember the food pyramid?

And I guess it's all true, we need each one of them but we shouldn't eat them together at the same time!

I enjoy different styles of fast food and I'm a strong believer that most of it is qualitative superior to most of the free-standing burger joints. But each one of them is forcing you to eat carbohydrates and protein at the same time!
???

While I'm writing this, I'm 100% convinced that this "new" train of thought (at least new for me) about food consumption is correct – it makes sense!

Unfortunately this is not the only rule you have to take care of.
There are a few more rules nearly as important as this one.
I come to them in a minute but let me first elaborate a bit more on the first rule.

Eat right 4 U'r kind

I'm sure you have heard of the famous non-carb diet. This diet stipulates that you should eat only meat in order to lose weight. (You are also allowed to eat vegetables and fruit beside meat)

The reasoning goes that if you don't eat any carbohydrates you will loose weight.

Meanwhile more and more voices are heard, warning of the detrimental effect it can have on your health.

Maybe I'm wrong - judge by yourself, but I never came across an overweight Vegetarian.

I know it's a funny thought but I reason that if you eat only meat you will lose weight but if you eat only vegetables you also lose weight?!?!?

Somehow it makes now sense to me that if you separate the two major food groups of protein and carbohydrates, you will not only speed up your digestion and live healthier, but you also may lose weight!

Please, I have to stress that I'm not a doctor, just a person with an active and inquisitive mind. The reasoning makes sense to me and following it, makes me feel better.

Here we go with all the rules I discovered:

Rule number one:

No protein and carbohydrate at the same meal!

Amylases is the enzyme that is used to digest starch / carbohydrates (works best in a neutral / alkaline environment - Ph 6.7 - 7).

Pepsin is the enzyme used to digest protein (works best in an acidic environment - Ph 1.5- 2).

Alkaline neutralizes acid.

If meat and starch is consumed during the same meal, the body will detect both food groups and excretes the appropriate enzymes. Consequently, digestion is hindered.
If this happens too often, the food can not be digested properly and possibly starts to ferment / rot. After an extended period inside your bowels it will be discarded into the large intestines.

The result is indigestion, chronic pains in the abdomen, a weakened immune system, followed by all kinds of ailments.

I still remember during my " healthy days" I would have a nice lunch, one of my favorites was beef goulash with spaetzle. Obviously - being a chef - home-made so it tasted exactly the way I loved it.
The moment I put my fork down I could feel the vibrations in my belly.
I thought maybe I'm hyper nervous...

Oh the taste buds in my mouth will miss this kind of food. Gone will be the times when I enjoyed a delicious sliced of veal "Zürichoise" with Roesti potatos. Just thinking about it - my mouth starts to water!
I used to have customers asking for some additional bread rolls to be able to clean their plates as the sauce is so delicious!
Gone!

Ragout Fin with butter Rice – Gone!

Sirloin steak "Café de Paris" with French fries – Gone!

Okay, okay, get out of it! Move on!

Here it is probably good to note that vegetables can be digested as well in an acid environment as in an alkaline environment.

Rules

Rule number two:

Don't combine acids and carbohydrates!

If you have cereals in the morning, make sure you don't put any orange juice to it.
Add no sour fruits and also no lemon juice!
It's again the same problem with carbohydrate-enzymes needing an alkaline/neutral environment to work properly and the disturbing influence of acids.

This means that a fresh orange juice is also out of the question if you're having bread for breakfast.

Rule number three:

Eat only one kind of protein at the same meal!

The explanation for this rule is that different kinds of proteins are digested in slightly different ways. For example meat needs a higher acidity during the beginning of digestion and less during the final stages.
Milk on the other hand needs a lower acidity at the beginning of digestion and a higher one at the end.
What follows is that, if both of them are consumed at the same time, both of them will not be digested properly!

Note: A couple of thousand years ago it was written in the Bible that you shouldn't cook the meat in its mother's milk.

Rule number four:

Eat melons alone!

The digestion of melons is extremely quick. Especially water melon. If melons are consumed with other foods, their digestion will be held up, resulting in fermentation and putrefaction.

Rule number five:

Forget about the desert!

The sweet stuff laying on top the other food you just have eaten can't be easily digested, interferes with the digestion of the previous food and creates - through fermentation - alcohol, vinegar and acetic acids.

Rule number six:

Red Wine is for meat and protein containing meals.

Beer is for starchy meals.

Don't ask me why but for some reason I know since a couple of years that I will pass on to the next chapter at the proud age of 92.

That is, if nothing unexpected happens .

(e.g. getting hit by a bus, crashing with an airplane, getting shot or falling off a tall tower)

I hope you enjoyed reading about my reasoning as much as I did discovering it.

If you have any comments about my conclusions, please feel free to drop me a line:

Alexanderwalz@didyoueverbook.com

Have a great rest of your life and remembered that today is the first day of it!

Hereafter one more time the rules without all the blah blah.

I have arranged them on different pages to enable you to cut them out and post them in convenient places to see and follow.

Rule number one:

! No protein and carbohydrate at the same meal!

Rule number two:

! **Don't combine acids and carbohydrates!**

Rule number three:

! Eat only one kind of protein at the same meal!

Rule number four:

! **Eat melons alone!**

Rule number five:

! **Forget about the desert!**

Rule number six:

Red Wine is for meat and protein containing meals.

Beer is for starchy meals.

www.ingramcontent.com/pod-product-compliance
Lightning Source LLC
Chambersburg PA
CBHW050337290526
45785CB00006B/2527